CARNIVORE DIET COOKBOOK

FOR BEGINNERS

Dr. Kimberly Carlos

TABLE OF CONTENT

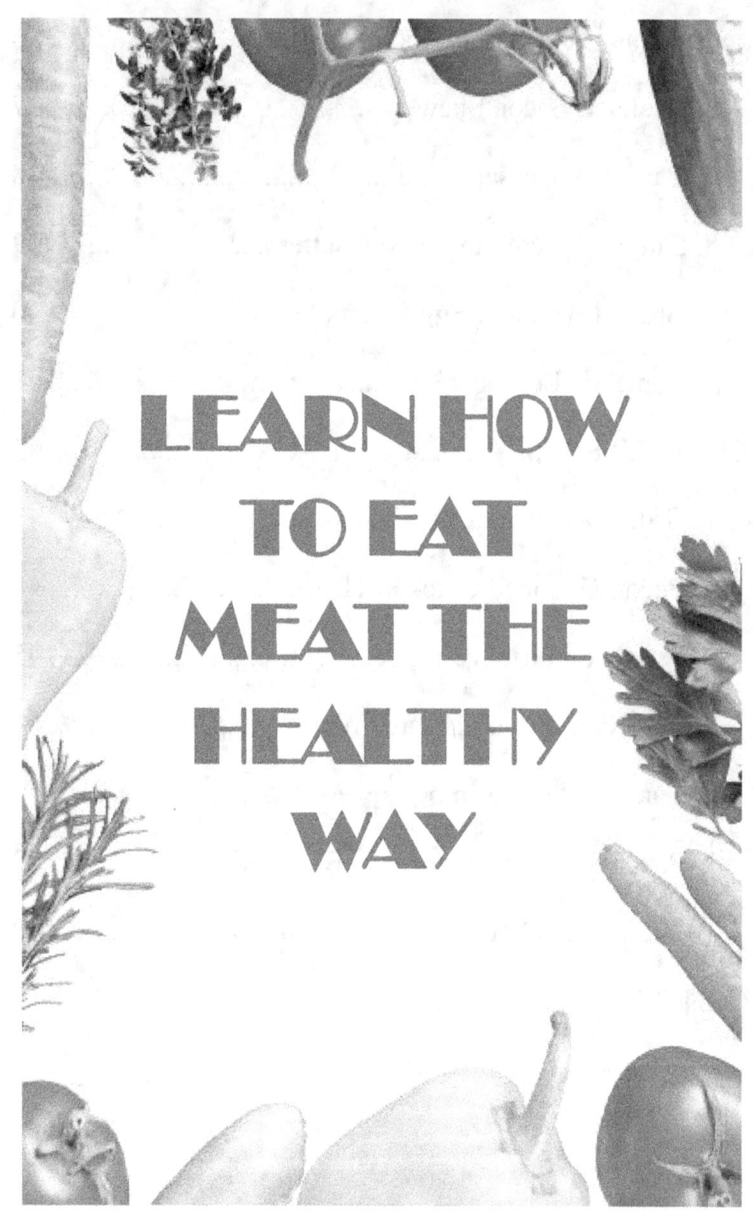
LEARN HOW
TO EAT
MEAT THE
HEALTHY
WAY

INTRODUCTION

In a world brimming with diverse dietary philosophies, the Carnivore Diet stands out as a distinctive and controversial approach that challenges conventional wisdom about nutrition.

Rooted in the consumption of animal products exclusively, this diet has sparked both intrigue and skepticism. As we delve into the fundamental principles and nuances of the Carnivore Diet, we embark on a journey that redefines our relationship with food and seeks to unlock the potential for optimal health.

Foundations of the Carnivore Diet

At its core, the Carnivore Diet is a form of the low-carbohydrate, high-fat (LCHF) diet that emphasizes the consumption of animal-based foods while eschewing plant-based products.

The cornerstone of this approach is the exclusion of fruits, vegetables, grains, and legumes, pushing boundaries beyond other low-carb diets like the ketogenic diet. The philosophy hinges on the belief that our ancestors predominantly subsisted on animal products, and by returning to this primal way of eating, we can unlock health benefits that extend far beyond weight management.

The Nutritional Paradigm Shift

For many accustomed to the nutritional status quo, the Carnivore Diet represents a radical shift. Traditionally, dietary guidelines advocate for a balanced plate comprising fruits, vegetables, grains, and lean proteins.

However, the Carnivore Diet challenges this paradigm, asserting that an exclusive focus on animal products provides all the essential nutrients our bodies require for optimal function. Proponents argue that this diet streamlines nutrition, eliminating potential allergens and anti-nutrients found in plant-based foods.

Understanding the Benefits

Advocates of the Carnivore Diet tout an array of potential benefits. From improved mental clarity and sustained energy levels to enhanced athletic performance and weight loss, adherents claim transformative changes in their overall well-being. Additionally, some individuals report relief from autoimmune conditions, digestive issues, and skin problems, attributing these improvements to the elimination of plant-based foods.

Critiques and Controversies

However, the Carnivore Diet is not without its critics. Skeptics raise concerns about potential nutrient deficiencies, the absence of dietary fiber, and the long-term health implications of excluding plant-based foods. The absence of large-scale, long-term studies on the Carnivore Diet adds to the ongoing debate within the scientific and medical communities.

As we embark on this exploration of the Carnivore Diet, it is essential to approach it with an open mind, considering both the success stories and the skepticism surrounding its efficacy. Over the course of our journey, we will delve into the science, anecdotal evidence, and the broader implications of adopting a diet that challenges conventional norms.

This comprehensive guide aims to provide a nuanced understanding of the Carnivore Diet, offering insights into its origins, the potential benefits and drawbacks, and practical considerations for those contemplating or currently navigating this unorthodox nutritional path. Whether you're a curious skeptic or an enthusiastic adopter, join us on this expedition into the world of the Carnivore Diet and discover the diverse perspectives that shape this intriguing approach to nutrition.

Let's take some delicious carnivore diet recipes for beginners...

CHAPTER ONE

Carnivore Diet Breakfast Recipes for Beginners

1. Carnivore Omelette

Ingredients:

- 3 large eggs

- 100g cooked and diced bacon

- 50g shredded cheddar cheese (optional)

- Salt and pepper to taste

- 1 tablespoon butter or ghee for cooking

Instructions:

1. In a bowl, whisk the eggs until well beaten.

2. Add the diced bacon to the eggs and mix thoroughly.

3. Heat the butter or ghee in a skillet over medium heat until melted.

4. Pour the egg and bacon mixture into the skillet.

5. Allow the edges to set, then gently lift them with a spatula

to let the uncooked egg flow underneath.

6. Once the omelette is mostly set, add the shredded cheddar cheese if desired.

7. Fold the omelette in half and cook for an additional minute until the cheese is melted and the eggs are fully cooked.

8. Season with salt and pepper to taste.

9. Serve hot and enjoy your carnivore-friendly omelette.

2. Carnivore Breakfast Skewers

Ingredients:

- 200g grilled sausage links

- 150g beef or pork liver, cooked and cubed

- 1 cup cherry tomatoes

- Salt and pepper to taste

Instructions:

1. Preheat your grill or stovetop grilling pan.

2. Cut the grilled sausage links into bite-sized pieces.

3. Thread the sausage pieces, cubed liver, and cherry tomatoes onto skewers, alternating them for a colorful presentation.

4. Grill the skewers until the sausage and liver are heated through and have a slight char.

5. Season with salt and pepper to taste.

6. Serve the carnivore breakfast skewers hot, providing a delicious and protein-packed start to your day.

3. Carnivore Steak and Eggs

Ingredients:

- 2 ribeye steaks (about 8 ounces each)

- Salt and pepper to taste

- 2 tablespoons butter or tallow for cooking

- 4 large eggs

Instructions:

1. Season the ribeye steaks generously with salt and pepper.

2. Heat the butter or tallow in a skillet over medium-high

heat.

3. Place the steaks in the skillet and cook to your preferred level of doneness (usually 3-4 minutes per side for medium-rare).

4. While the steaks are cooking, fry the eggs in a separate pan.

5. Once the steaks are done, transfer them to a plate and let them rest for a few minutes.

6. Serve the ribeye steaks with fried eggs on top, creating a protein-packed and flavorful carnivore breakfast.

4. Carnivore Bacon and Egg Cups

Ingredients:

- 6 slices of bacon

- 6 large eggs

- Salt and pepper to taste

- Fresh herbs for garnish (optional)

Instructions:

1. Preheat your oven to 375°F (190°C).

2. Line a muffin tin with bacon slices, creating a cup shape.

3. Crack an egg into each bacon cup.

4. Season with salt and pepper.

5. Bake in the preheated oven for 15-20 minutes or until the egg whites are set.

6. Garnish with fresh herbs if desired.

7. Serve these bacon and egg cups hot for a carnivore-friendly breakfast.

5. Carnivore Salmon and Cream Cheese Rolls

Ingredients:

- Smoked salmon slices

- 100g cream cheese

- Fresh chives, chopped, for garnish

Instructions:

1. Lay out the smoked salmon slices.

2. Spread a thin layer of cream cheese over each slice.

3. Roll up the salmon slices with the cream cheese inside.

4. Secure with toothpicks if needed.

5. Garnish with chopped fresh chives.

6. Serve these delicious salmon and cream cheese rolls as a unique and satisfying carnivore breakfast option.

6. Carnivore Sausage and Cheese Omelette

Ingredients:

- 4 large eggs

- 2 carnivore-friendly sausages, cooked and crumbled

- 1/2 cup shredded cheddar cheese

- Salt and pepper to taste

- Butter for cooking

Instructions:

1. In a bowl, whisk the eggs and season with salt and pepper.

2. Heat butter in a skillet over medium heat.

3. Pour the whisked eggs into the skillet, allowing them to set slightly around the edges.

4. Sprinkle the crumbled sausage and shredded cheddar cheese over one half of the omelette.

5. Fold the other half of the omelette over the sausage and cheese.

6. Continue cooking until the cheese is melted, and the omelette is cooked through.

7. Serve this hearty sausage and cheese omelette for a filling carnivore breakfast.

7. Carnivore Avocado and Bacon Bowl

Ingredients:

- 2 avocados, halved and pitted

- 4 slices of cooked bacon, crumbled

- Salt and pepper to taste

- Fresh parsley, chopped, for garnish (optional)

Instructions:

1. Scoop out a bit of the avocado flesh to create a larger well in each half.

2. Season the avocado halves with salt and pepper.

3. Fill each avocado half with crumbled bacon.

4. Garnish with chopped fresh parsley if desired.

5. Serve these avocado and bacon bowls for a simple yet satisfying carnivore breakfast.

8. Carnivore Steak and Eggs Skillet

Ingredients:

- 2 ribeye steaks

- Salt and black pepper to taste

- 4 eggs

- Butter for cooking

Instructions:

1. Season the ribeye steaks with salt and black pepper.

2. Heat butter in a skillet over medium-high heat.

3. Cook the steaks to your preferred doneness.

4. In the same skillet, crack the eggs around the steaks and cook them to your liking.

5. Serve the steaks with eggs for a protein-packed carnivore breakfast.

9. Carnivore Breakfast Burger
Ingredients:

- 2 beef patties

- Salt and pepper to taste

- 2 slices of cheese (optional)

- Lettuce leaves for wrapping

Instructions:

1. Season the beef patties with salt and pepper.

2. Cook the patties to your desired doneness.

3. If desired, place a slice of cheese on each patty and let it melt.

4. Use lettuce leaves to wrap the beef patties, creating a

breakfast burger.

10. Carnivore Salmon and Cream Cheese Roll-Ups

Ingredients:

- Smoked salmon slices

- Cream cheese

- Capers (optional)

- Chopped chives (optional)

Instructions:

1. Spread a layer of cream cheese on each smoked salmon slice.

2. Place capers and chopped chives along one edge of the salmon slices.

3. Roll up the salmon slices, starting from the edge with capers and chives.

4. Secure the rolls with toothpicks if needed.

5. Enjoy these savory salmon and cream cheese roll-ups for a refreshing carnivore breakfast.

CHAPTER TWO

Carnivore Diet Lunch Recipes for Beginners

11. Carnivore Beef and Bacon Skewers

Ingredients:

- Beef chunks

- Bacon strips

- Salt and black pepper to taste

Instructions:

1. Preheat a grill or grill pan.

2. Thread beef chunks and bacon strips onto skewers, alternating between them.

3. Season the skewers with salt and black pepper.

4. Grill the skewers until the beef is cooked to your liking and the bacon is crispy.

5. Serve these flavorful beef and bacon skewers for a satisfying carnivore lunch.

12. Carnivore Chicken Thighs with Herb Butter

Ingredients:

- Chicken thighs

- Salt and dried herbs (rosemary, thyme, or your choice)

- Butter

Instructions:

1. Preheat the oven to 400°F (200°C).

2. Season chicken thighs with salt and dried herbs.

3. Place chicken thighs on a baking sheet.

4. Dot each thigh with a small amount of butter.

5. Bake in the oven until the chicken is thoroughly cooked and the skin is crispy.

6. Enjoy these juicy and herb-infused carnivore chicken thighs for lunch.

13. Carnivore Egg and Ground Beef Scramble

Ingredients:

- 1 pound ground beef

- 6 eggs

- Salt and pepper to taste

Instructions:

1. In a skillet, cook 1 pound of ground beef until browned and cooked through.

2. Crack 6 eggs into the skillet with the cooked beef.

3. Scramble the eggs with the beef, ensuring they are fully cooked.

4. Season with salt and pepper.

5. Serve this hearty and protein-packed egg and ground beef scramble for a quick and delicious carnivore lunch.

14. Carnivore Shrimp Stir-Fry

Ingredients:

- 1 pound shrimp

- Beef tallow or preferred animal fat for cooking

- Salt and garlic powder to taste

Instructions:

1. Heat beef tallow or your chosen fat in a skillet.

2. Add 1 pound of shrimp to the skillet and cook until they turn pink and opaque.

3. Season with salt and garlic powder.

4. Stir-fry until the shrimp are fully cooked.

5. Enjoy this carnivore shrimp stir-fry as a flavorful and low-carb lunch option.

15. Carnivore Lamb Chops

Ingredients:

- Lamb chops (quantity as desired)

- Salt and rosemary for seasoning

Instructions:

1. Preheat the grill or oven.

2. Season lamb chops with salt and rosemary.

3. Grill or bake the lamb chops until they reach your desired level of doneness.

4. Allow the chops to rest before serving.

5. Delight in the rich and succulent flavors of carnivore lamb chops for a satisfying lunch.

16. Carnivore Beef Liver Sauté

Ingredients:

- 1 pound beef liver

- Beef tallow for cooking

- Salt and pepper to taste

Instructions:

1. Slice 1 pound of beef liver into thin strips.

2. Heat beef tallow in a skillet.

3. Sauté the beef liver strips until browned on both sides.

4. Season with salt and pepper to taste.

5. Serve this nutrient-dense beef liver sauté as a powerful addition to your carnivore lunch.

17. Carnivore Chicken Thighs

Ingredients:

- Chicken thighs (quantity as desired)

- Duck fat or preferred animal fat for cooking

- Garlic powder and thyme for seasoning

Instructions:

1. Preheat the oven.

2. Rub chicken thighs with garlic powder and thyme.

3. Place the thighs on a baking sheet and drizzle with duck fat or your chosen fat.

4. Roast in the oven until the chicken reaches an internal temperature of 165°F (74°C).

5. Enjoy these juicy and flavorful carnivore chicken thighs for a satisfying lunch.

18. Carnivore Ribeye Steak

Ingredients:

- Ribeye steak (quantity as desired)

- Salt and pepper to taste

- Beef tallow for cooking

Instructions:

1. Preheat a cast-iron skillet with beef tallow.

2. Season the ribeye steak with salt and pepper.

3. Sear the steak in the hot skillet until it reaches your preferred level of doneness.

4. Allow it to rest for a few minutes before slicing and

serving.

5. Enjoy this simple and delicious carnivore ribeye steak for a hearty lunch.

19. Carnivore Egg Drop Soup

Ingredients:

- Beef or chicken bone broth (2 cups)

- Ground beef or pork (1/2 pound)

- Eggs (2)

- Salt and pepper to taste

- Chopped fresh herbs (optional)

Instructions:

1. In a pot, heat the bone broth until simmering.

2. Add ground beef or pork and cook until fully cooked.

3. Crack the eggs into the simmering broth and stir gently to create egg ribbons.

4. Season with salt and pepper to taste.

5. Optionally, garnish with chopped fresh herbs before serving.

20. Carnivore Bacon-Wrapped Chicken Thighs

Ingredients:

- Chicken thighs (4)

- Bacon strips (8)

- Salt and pepper to taste

Instructions:

1. Preheat the oven to 400°F (200°C).

2. Season the chicken thighs with salt and pepper.

3. Wrap each chicken thigh with two bacon strips, ensuring they are fully covered.

4. Place the bacon-wrapped chicken thighs on a baking sheet.

5. Bake in the preheated oven for about 25-30 minutes or until the bacon is crispy and the chicken is fully cooked.

6. Allow it to cool for a few minutes before serving.

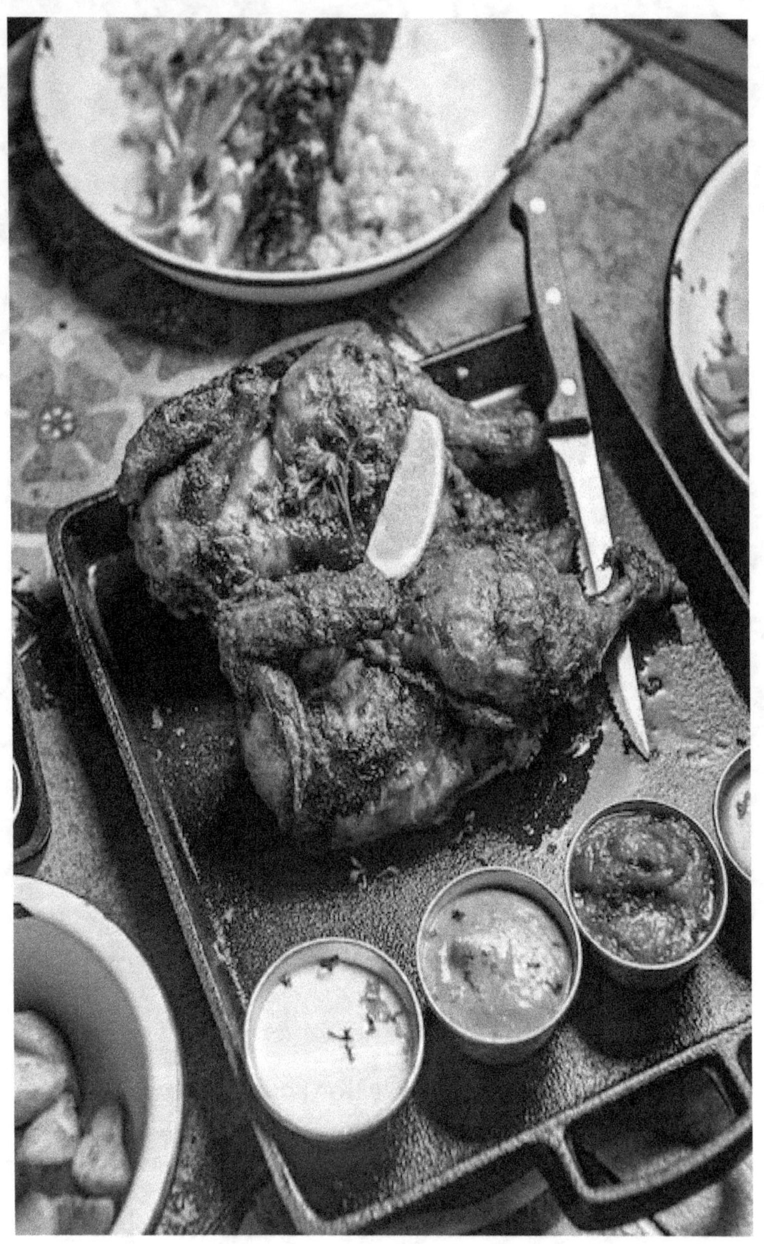

CHAPTER FOUR

Bone Broth Recipes for Meat Lovers

1. Classic Beef Bone Broth

Ingredients:

- Beef bones (2-3 lbs, marrow and knuckle bones)

- Water (16 cups)

- Apple cider vinegar (2 tablespoons)

- Onion (1, quartered)

- Carrots (2, chopped)

- Celery (2 stalks, chopped)

- Garlic cloves (4, smashed)

- Fresh parsley (a handful)

- Bay leaves (2)

- Salt and pepper to taste

Instructions:

1. Preheat the oven to 400°F (200°C). Place beef bones on a

baking sheet and roast for about 30 minutes, turning once.

2. Transfer the roasted bones to a large stockpot. Add water, apple cider vinegar, and bring to a boil.

3. Skim off any foam that rises to the top. Reduce heat to a simmer.

4. Add onion, carrots, celery, garlic, parsley, bay leaves, salt, and pepper.

5. Simmer the broth on low heat for at least 8 hours or up to 24 hours.

6. Strain the broth, discarding solids. Allow it to cool, then refrigerate or freeze.

2. Savory Chicken Bone Broth

Ingredients:

- Chicken bones (2-3 lbs, including backs and necks)

- Water (16 cups)

- Apple cider vinegar (2 tablespoons)

- Onion (1, quartered)

- Carrots (2, chopped)

- Celery (2 stalks, chopped)

- Thyme (1 tablespoon, fresh or dried)

- Rosemary (1 tablespoon, fresh or dried)

- Bay leaves (2)

- Salt and pepper to taste

Instructions:

1. Place chicken bones in a large stockpot. Add water and apple cider vinegar, and bring to a boil.

2. Skim off any foam that rises to the top. Reduce heat to a simmer.

3. Add onion, carrots, celery, thyme, rosemary, bay leaves, salt, and pepper.

4. Simmer the broth on low heat for at least 4-6 hours.

5. Strain the broth, discarding solids. Allow it to cool, then refrigerate or freeze.

3. Grilled Ribeye Steak Salad

Ingredients:

- Ribeye steak (1, thick-cut)

- Salt and pepper to taste

- Olive oil (2 tablespoons)

- Mixed salad greens (2 cups)

- Cherry tomatoes (1 cup, halved)

- Red onion (1/2, thinly sliced)

- Balsamic vinaigrette dressing (to taste)

Instructions:

1. Season the ribeye steak with salt and pepper.

2. Preheat the grill or grill pan to medium-high heat.

3. Brush the steak with olive oil and grill for 4-5 minutes per side (medium-rare), or to your desired doneness.

4. Let the steak rest for a few minutes before slicing it thinly.

5. In a large bowl, combine the mixed salad greens, cherry

tomatoes, and red onion.

6. Top the salad with sliced grilled ribeye.

7. Drizzle with balsamic vinaigrette and toss gently. Serve and enjoy.

4. Bacon-Wrapped Chicken Thighs

Ingredients:

- Chicken thighs (4, boneless and skinless)

- Bacon strips (8)

- Garlic powder (1 teaspoon)

- Paprika (1 teaspoon)

- Salt and pepper to taste

Instructions:

1. Preheat the oven to 400°F (200°C).

2. Season the chicken thighs with garlic powder, paprika, salt, and pepper.

3. Wrap each chicken thigh with two bacon strips, ensuring

they're securely wrapped.

4. Place the wrapped chicken thighs on a baking sheet lined with parchment paper.

5. Bake for 25-30 minutes or until the chicken is cooked through and the bacon is crispy.

6. Remove from the oven and let it rest for a few minutes before serving.

5. Salmon Avocado Lettuce Wraps

Ingredients:

- Salmon fillets (2, skinless)

- Olive oil (2 tablespoons)

- Lemon juice (1 tablespoon)

- Salt and pepper to taste

- Iceberg lettuce leaves (8)

- Avocado (1, sliced)

- Cucumber (1, julienned)

- Fresh dill (for garnish)

Instructions:

1. Preheat the oven to 400°F (200°C).

2. Place salmon fillets on a baking sheet. Drizzle with olive oil and lemon juice. Season with salt and pepper.

3. Bake for 12-15 minutes or until the salmon flakes easily with a fork.

4. While the salmon is baking, prepare lettuce leaves and toppings.

5. Flake the cooked salmon and assemble lettuce wraps with salmon, sliced avocado, and julienned cucumber.

6. Garnish with fresh dill and serve.

Certainly! Here are two more Carnivore Diet lunch recipes for beginners:

6. Beef and Bacon Skewers

Ingredients:

- Beef chunks (1 pound, sirloin or ribeye)

- Bacon strips (1/2 pound, cut into squares)

- Salt and black pepper to taste

- Wooden skewers (pre-soaked in water)

Instructions:

1. Preheat the grill or broiler.

2. Season beef chunks with salt and pepper.

3. Thread beef and bacon alternately onto the skewers.

4. Grill or broil for 5-7 minutes per side or until cooked to your liking.

5. Serve immediately and enjoy the flavorful combination of beef and bacon.

7. Carnivore Caesar Salad

Ingredients:

- Romaine lettuce (1 head, chopped)

- Grilled chicken breast (2 breasts, sliced)

- Parmesan cheese (1/2 cup, shaved)

- Caesar dressing (1/4 cup)

- Black pepper to taste

Instructions:

1. In a large bowl, combine chopped Romaine lettuce and grilled chicken slices.

2. Drizzle Caesar dressing over the salad and toss until well-coated.

3. Top with shaved Parmesan cheese and sprinkle with black pepper.

4. Toss again and serve this carnivore-friendly Caesar salad.

8. Salmon Fillet with Lemon Butter

Ingredients:

- Salmon fillets (2, skin-on)

- Salt and black pepper to taste

- Butter (2 tablespoons)

- Lemon juice (1 tablespoon)

- Fresh parsley (chopped, for garnish)

Instructions:

1. Preheat the oven to 400°F (200°C).

2. Season the salmon fillets with salt and pepper.

3. In an oven-safe skillet, melt butter over medium heat.

4. Place the salmon fillets in the skillet, skin-side down.

5. Sear for 2-3 minutes, then transfer the skillet to the preheated oven.

6. Bake for 10-12 minutes or until the salmon is cooked through.

7. Drizzle lemon juice over the salmon, garnish with chopped parsley, and serve.

9. Ground Beef and Egg Scramble

Ingredients:

- Ground beef (1/2 pound)

- Eggs (4)

- Salt and black pepper to taste

- Ghee or tallow (2 tablespoons)

Instructions:

1. In a skillet, heat ghee or tallow over medium heat.

2. Add ground beef to the skillet and cook until browned.

3. Crack the eggs into the skillet and scramble them with the cooked beef.

4. Season with salt and pepper to taste.

5. Continue cooking until the eggs are fully scrambled and cooked.

6. Serve this protein-packed beef and egg scramble hot.

10. Chicken Liver Pâté

Ingredients:

- Chicken livers (1/2 pound)

- Butter (4 tablespoons)

- Garlic cloves (2, minced)

- Salt and black pepper to taste

Instructions:

1. In a skillet, melt butter over medium heat.

2. Add minced garlic and chicken livers to the skillet.

3. Cook the chicken livers until they are no longer pink inside.

4. Transfer the cooked livers and garlic to a food processor.

5. Blend until smooth, season with salt and pepper.

6. Refrigerate the pâté for at least 2 hours before serving.

7. Spread on cucumber slices or eat as a dip.

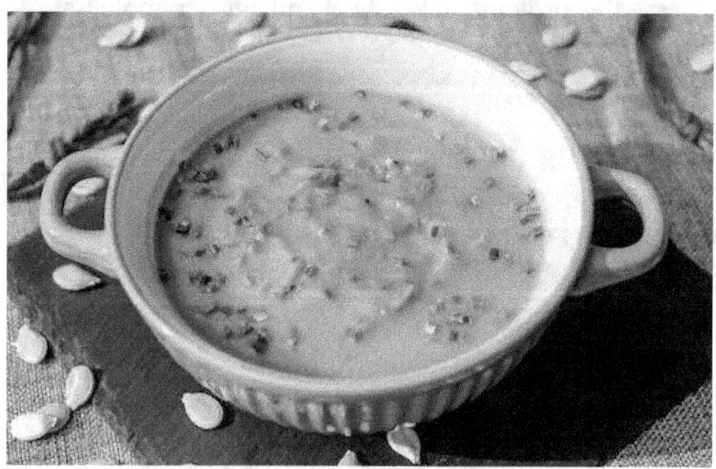

CHAPTER FIVE

1. Grilled Ribeye Steak with Garlic Butter

Ingredients:

- Ribeye steaks (2, about 1 pound each)

- Salt and black pepper to taste

- Olive oil (2 tablespoons)

- Butter (4 tablespoons)

- Garlic cloves (4, minced)

- Fresh parsley (chopped, for garnish)

Instructions:

1. Preheat your grill to high heat.

2. Rub the ribeye steaks with olive oil and season generously with salt and pepper.

3. Place the steaks on the hot grill and cook for 4-5 minutes per side for medium-rare, or adjust based on your desired doneness.

4. In a small saucepan, melt butter over medium heat.

5. Add minced garlic to the melted butter and sauté for 1-2 minutes until fragrant.

6. Pour the garlic butter over the grilled ribeye steaks.

7. Garnish with chopped parsley and let the steaks rest for a few minutes before serving.

2. Bacon-Wrapped Chicken Thighs

Ingredients:

- Chicken thighs (4, boneless and skinless)

- Salt and black pepper to taste

- Smoked paprika (1 teaspoon)

- Garlic powder (1 teaspoon)

- Bacon strips (8)

- Olive oil (1 tablespoon)

- Fresh thyme leaves (for garnish)

Instructions:

1. Preheat your oven to 400°F (200°C).

2. Season the chicken thighs with salt, pepper, smoked paprika, and garlic powder.

3. Wrap each chicken thigh with 2 strips of bacon, securing with toothpicks if needed.

4. Heat olive oil in an oven-safe skillet over medium-high heat.

5. Sear the bacon-wrapped chicken thighs for 2-3 minutes on each side until the bacon is golden brown.

6. Transfer the skillet to the preheated oven and bake for 20-25 minutes or until the chicken is cooked through.

7. Garnish with fresh thyme leaves before serving.

6. Pan-Seared Ribeye Steak

Ingredients:

- Ribeye steak (1 inch thick)

- Salt and black pepper to taste

- Butter (2 tablespoons)

- Fresh thyme (a few sprigs)

- Garlic cloves (2, smashed)

Instructions:

1. Season the ribeye steak generously with salt and black pepper.

2. Heat a cast-iron skillet over medium-high heat.

3. Add butter, fresh thyme, and smashed garlic cloves to the skillet.

4. Place the ribeye steak in the skillet and sear for 3-4 minutes on each side for medium-rare (adjust cooking time based on your preference).

5. Baste the steak with the melted butter, thyme, and garlic during cooking.

6. Let the steak rest for a few minutes before slicing and serving.

7. Carnivore Burger Lettuce Wraps

Ingredients:

- Ground beef (1 pound)

- Salt and black pepper to taste

- Cheese slices (optional)

- Iceberg lettuce leaves (for wrapping)

- Condiments and toppings of choice (mayonnaise, mustard, pickles)

Instructions:

1. Season the ground beef with salt and black pepper and form into burger patties.

2. Heat a grill or skillet over medium-high heat.

3. Cook the burger patties for 3-4 minutes per side or until they reach your desired level of doneness.

4. If desired, place a slice of cheese on top of each patty and let it melt.

5. Wrap the burger patties in iceberg lettuce leaves.

6. Add your favorite condiments and toppings.

8. Garlic Butter Shrimp Skewers

Ingredients:

- Shrimp, peeled and deveined (1 pound)

- Butter (4 tablespoons, melted)

- Garlic powder (1 teaspoon)

- Salt and black pepper to taste

- Fresh parsley, chopped (for garnish)

Instructions:

1. Preheat a grill or grill pan over medium-high heat.

2. In a bowl, mix melted butter, garlic powder, salt, and black pepper.

3. Thread the shrimp onto skewers and brush them generously with the garlic butter mixture.

4. Grill the shrimp skewers for 2-3 minutes on each side or until they turn opaque.

5. Remove from the grill, garnish with fresh parsley, and serve.

9. Bacon-Wrapped Asparagus Bundles
Ingredients:

- Asparagus spears (1 bunch)

- Bacon slices (1 slice per asparagus spear)

- Olive oil (1 tablespoon)

- Salt and black pepper to taste

Instructions:

1. Preheat the oven to 400°F (200°C).

2. Trim the tough ends of the asparagus and divide them into bundles.

3. Wrap each asparagus bundle with a slice of bacon.

4. Place the bundles on a baking sheet, drizzle with olive oil, and season with salt and black pepper.

5. Bake in the preheated oven for 20-25 minutes or until the bacon is crispy.

10. Carnivore Omelette with Ground Beef
Ingredients:

- Ground beef (1/2 pound)

- Eggs (3)

- Salt and black pepper to taste

- Olive oil or butter for cooking

- Optional: Cheese slices (if allowed in your carnivore diet)

Instructions:

1. In a skillet, cook the ground beef until browned. Season with salt and black pepper.

2. In a bowl, beat the eggs and season with salt and black pepper.

3. Heat olive oil or butter in a separate pan over medium heat.

4. Pour the beaten eggs into the pan and let them set slightly.

5. Add the cooked ground beef to one half of the omelette.

6. If desired, place cheese slices on top of the ground beef.

7. Fold the omelette in half, covering the ground beef and cheese.

8. Cook for an additional 1-2 minutes until the cheese melts, and the omelette is cooked to your liking.

CONCLUSION

In conclusion, this Carnivore Diet Cookbook for Beginners is not just a collection of recipes; it's a guide to transforming your eating habits and embracing a lifestyle centered around nutrient-dense, animal-based foods.

As you journey through these pages, you've explored the simplicity and richness of the carnivore diet, discovering the myriad ways to savor meat, seafood, and other carnivore-friendly ingredients.

This cookbook is more than a culinary adventure; it's a commitment to optimal health and well-being. By following the recipes and principles outlined here, you're not only satisfying your taste buds but also providing your body with the essential nutrients it craves.

You've witnessed the versatility of carnivore cooking, from juicy steaks to savory stews and delightful skewers.

Embracing the carnivore diet isn't just about what you eat; it's a holistic approach to nourishing your body and mind. You've learned about the potential benefits of this diet, from improved energy levels and mental clarity to weight management and enhanced athletic performance. The carnivore lifestyle is not just a trend; it's a sustainable and ancestral way of eating that reconnects us with the foods that our bodies have evolved to thrive on.

As you savor the delicious recipes crafted for beginners, remember that this is just the beginning of your carnivore journey. Use this cookbook as a foundation to explore and experiment, adapting the recipes to suit your taste preferences and nutritional needs. Whether you're seeking simplicity or culinary creativity, the carnivore diet offers a spectrum of possibilities.

Thank you for joining this culinary exploration of the carnivore diet. May this cookbook empower you to take charge of your health, relish the joy of preparing and enjoying wholesome meals, and embark on a transformative journey toward a vibrant and carnivorous life.

Cheers to your health, happiness, and the flavorful world of the carnivore diet!

www.ingramcontent.com/pod-product-compliance
Lightning Source LLC
Chambersburg PA
CBHW070732260726

48660CB00007B/2812